Penguin Books

Physical Fitness: 5BX

The

5BX Plan

for Physical Fitness
for Men

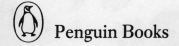

Penguin Books

PENGUIN BOOKS

Published by the Penguin Group
Penguin Books Ltd, 27 Wrights Lane, London W8 5TZ, England
Penguin Putnam Inc., 375 Hudson Street, New York, New York 10014, USA
Penguin Books Australia Ltd, Ringwood, Victoria, Australia
Penguin Books Canada Ltd, 10 Alcorn Avenue, Toronto, Ontario, Canada M4V 3B2
Penguin Books (NZ) Ltd, Private Bag 102902, NSMC, Auckland, New Zealand

Penguin Books Ltd, Registered Offices: Harmondsworth, Middlesex, England

5BX first published by the RCAF 1958
XBX first published by the RCAF 1960
Published in one volume in Penguin Books 1964
This separate volume published 1986
20 19 18 17 16 15 14 13

Photographs by Colin Thomas
Crown copyright © Queen's Printer, Canada, 1958, 1960
Reproduced by permission
All rights reserved

Printed in England by Clays Ltd, St Ives plc
Set in Linotron Ehrhardt

Contents

Foreword

This is an age in which, even in the country, more and more people go everywhere on wheels. Keeping fit has become a universal problem. Though they may not be willing to spend time and money at a gymnasium and have no ambitions in the sphere of the 'body beautiful', very many people are nevertheless worried today about their figures and their general state of health.

The system of exercises detailed in this book presents an exceedingly simple answer to the problem. These plans were developed by the Royal Canadian Air Force in order to keep personnel at a peak of physical fitness, ready to face sudden demands for energy after long periods of inactivity. When they were made available to the general public, the two booklets of exercises rapidly became bestsellers all over North America. Their publication in Penguins will enable them to reach an even wider audience.

These exercises are specially designed for those who are pressed for time, whose work is mainly sedentary, and who have neither the space nor the taste for formal games or walks; for city-dwellers (in particular) who, even if they hardly ever go to the shops without a car, may occasionally have to sprint for a bus or climb stairs when the lift is out of order; and for those who are becoming aware of 'middle-aged spread' or of the strain of work, but are disinclined to take very strong action.

The 5BX plan, as these exercises are called, is graded progressively and the performer is not expected to go beyond the simpler movements at the beginning of the course until he or she can do them without difficulty in the time set. The pace of progress and the degree of fitness are entirely up to the performer. In this way it has been proved that adequate fitness can be achieved by easy stages, in very little space and without exaggerated exertion, at the cost of only a few minutes each day. Above all this system does not reach too high. It aims to provide the right degree of fitness for all normal purposes, without arousing any anxiety about Olympic standards of training.

The 5BX is ideal for anyone who simply wants to get fit, look fit, feel fit, and stay fit.

Acknowledgements

The R.C.A.F. acknowledges the contribution made to the preparation of the 5BX Pamphlet by W. A. R. Orban, Ph.D., Canadian physical education experts, and R.C.A.F. medical advisers.

Introduction

Why You Should Be Fit

Research has shown that the physically fit person is able to withstand fatigue for longer periods than the unfit; that the physically fit person is better equipped to tolerate physical stress; that the physically fit person has a stronger and more efficient heart; and that there is a relationship between good mental alertness, absence of nervous tension, and physical fitness.

Remember that:

(1) weak stomach muscles cause sagging abdomens; and
(2) weak back muscles are a major cause of back pain.

There are countless reasons for being fit. *You* know how you feel. *Everyone* knows how you look. Regular exercise can improve your sense of well-being and your appearance. Fitness is necessary for the fullest enjoyment of living.

Weight Control

The major purpose of weight control is to reduce the amount of fat on the body and to increase the amount of muscle. It is, in reality, a programme of fat control rather than weight control. This control can be exerted only by coupling a sensible dietary programme with a regular, balanced programme of exercise.

When we eat, the food is used, stored, or discarded. The body stores fuel, or calories, as fat. The more fuel we consume, and the less of it we use, then the more of it that is stored in the body in the form of fat. The human body is not like a car's petrol tank that will overflow when full. Our bodies accept all the calories that we put into them, and store those which we do not use.

For example, if you eat food that has a value of 3,000 calories and use only 2,600 of them in your activity, then the remaining 400 calories are stored in the body. Every time you accumulate about 4,000 of these calories you will notice an extra pound of weight on the scales.

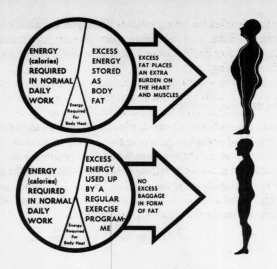

When you exercise you burn calories. Energy used in this way will result in muscle development. As muscle is slightly heavier than fat, you may very well notice an increase in your weight rather than a reduction. However it must be stressed that this muscle weight is useful weight and will improve the way you look and feel.

Research has shown clearly that the most effective way of taking off weight and keeping it off is through a programme which combines exercise and diet.

Live To Be Fit and Be Fit To Live

This book is concerned primarily with the habits of exercise and diet as steps on the road to fitness. Many more ways and means exist which can become habits that will also contribute to this goal. Try to make some of these a part of your daily living and you will soon find that without conscious effort, or extra 'work', you are gaining many benefits.

Walking is an excellent exercise if done at a faster pace than a slow shuffle. If you use public transport, do not use the nearest or most convenient stop, but get on or off a few streets away and walk briskly. Walk to the corner shop or post box rather than use your car. At every opportunity, walk rather than ride. Climb a few flights of stairs instead of using the lift or escalator.

Use your muscles for lifting objects when you are able, rather than pushing them. Even an everyday practice like drying yourself with a towel after bathing can become a fitness activity. Rub down briskly rather than dabbing.

While sitting at a desk or table you can aid posture and tone up muscles. Sit tall with your back straight; do not slump with round back and shoulders, and head forward. To tone up the shoulder girdle and arm muscles: sit erect, place hands on desk, palms down, elbows bent, and press down, trying to lift body from chair. Hold the pressure for a few seconds. Repeat two or three times a day.

When standing, sitting, or lying, tense the muscles of the abdomen and hold for about six seconds. Do this a few times each day. Constantly think of how you look, and walk tall and sit tall, always attempting to maintain a good postural position.

Rest, Relaxation, and Revitalization

It is just as important that your body receives adequate rest as it is that it be exercised. Sleep requirements vary from person to person and each person is his own best judge of these needs. The important thing is to awake refreshed and revitalized. A few tips on getting the most from your bedtime hours:

(1) keep the room as dark as possible;
(2) do not take your problems to bed with you – if you must think, think calm, restful thoughts;
(3) mild exercise before retiring may be helpful;
(4) if you are hungry, have a light snack or a warm, non-stimulating beverage.

Relaxation, both mental and physical, is becoming more and more essential in the fast moving, hurly-burly world in which we live. Many emotional tensions are reflected in physical tensions, both organic and muscular.

You can consciously reduce both forms of tension. Physically you can learn to relax muscle groups. A simple illustration is this: hold your hands in front of you, tighten up the muscles of the forearms so that the hands and fingers are straight, abruptly relax them so that the hands fall limply. Try this with other muscles – tighten – then relax. Stretch, writhe, and wriggle yourself into a relaxed state.

For mental relaxation try consciously to think pleasant and restful thoughts, ignoring for a while the troubles of the day. Healthy forms of recreation (picnics, golf, etc.) are fine ways to release not only the physical tensions, but some of the mental ones as well.

Exercise and the Heart

There are many misconceptions about exercise and its effect upon the heart. 'Exercise is harmful.' Nonsense. There is no evidence to support this contention. There is a large body of opinion which holds that exercise, appropriate to age and physical condition, continued through your life span, will help to reduce the possibility of heart and blood vessel disease. Exercise, in mild form of course, is recommended as part of the recuperative phase in cases of heart or coronary disease. Evidence is also on hand that indicates exercise is beneficial to the function of the cardio-vascular system.

A healthy heart can obtain many benefits from a good conditioning programme. Research has shown that the heart of a trained person has a smaller acceleration of pulse rate under stress, and that it returns more rapidly to its normal rate afterwards than that of an untrained person; that it pumps more blood per beat at rest, and that it can pump more during exercise; that it has more richly developed small blood vessels supplying the heart muscle and that it functions more efficiently. An efficient cardio-vascular system means a better supply of food and oxygen to the muscles (as blood is the carrier of these items) and a quicker recuperation after exertion, be it work, play, or exercise.

A cautionary note: persons over thirty-five years of age, and anyone who suspects that they may have something wrong with their heart, should have a thorough medical examination before engaging in a vigorous exercise programme. Experts have noted that a heart already injured by disease will suffer extra abuse through extreme forms of exercise. Sudden violent exertion after a period of inactivity is to be avoided.

Exercise, Strength, and Endurance

The strength and endurance of the body can be increased through regular exercise. Such improvements are primarily localized in the muscles and organs which are exercised – one cannot strengthen the arms and shoulders by exercising the legs. To improve the condition of all muscles one must undertake a programme which will provide them all with work.

The strength of a muscle is measured by the amount of force that that muscle can exert and is dependent upon the size and number of muscle fibres that can be brought into action at any one time and the frequency of the nerve impulses to them.

Endurance is concerned with the ability to repeat an action over and over again, or to sustain a muscular contraction.

Since the fuel for muscular contraction is carried in the blood, endurance is chiefly dependent upon the functioning of the cardio-respiratory system (heart, blood vessels, and lungs) – that is, the ability of the body to transport food and oxygen to the muscles, and waste products away from them, efficiently.

The human body requires proper use to function efficiently and endure. The body is very different from a machine that wears out with use. Most persons have noted how the muscles of an arm or a leg in a cast become smaller and weaker the longer the arm or leg remains so encased. While this is a dramatic example it is in effect what happens to the muscles of the body in a milder way when these muscles are not used enough. Exercise over and above the normal demands of daily living is essential to the development of an efficient, strong, and durable body. The resultant more pleasing appearance and sense of well-being are added benefits that cannot be overlooked.

Caution – before you start

If you have any doubt as to your capability to undertake this programme, *see your medical adviser*. You should not perform fast, vigorous, or highly competitive physical activity without gradually developing, and continuously maintaining, an adequate level of physical fitness, particularly if you are over the age of 30.

The 5BX Plan for Men

Physical Fitness

The human body is made up mainly of bone, muscle, and fat. Some 639 different muscles account for about 45 per cent of the body weight. Each of these muscles has four distinct and measurable qualities which are of interest to us:

(1) it can produce force which can be measured as strength of muscle;

(2) it can store energy which permits it to work for extended periods of time independent of circulation – this is generally referred to as *muscular endurance*;

(3) it can shorten at varying rates. This is called *speed of contraction*;

(4) it can be stretched and will recoil. This is called the *elasticity of muscle*.

The combination of these four qualities of muscle is referred to as *muscular power*.

If muscles are to function efficiently, they must be continually supplied with energy fuel. This is accomplished by the blood which carries the energy fuel from lungs and digestive system to the muscles. The blood is forced through the blood vessels by the heart. The combined capacity to supply energy fuels to the working muscles is called *organic power*.

The capacity and efficiency with which your body can function depends on the degree of development of both your muscular and organic power through regular exercise. However, the level to which you can develop these powers is influenced by such factors as the type of body you have, the food you eat, presence or absence of disease, rest and sleep. You are physically fit only when you have adequately developed your muscular and organic power to perform with the highest possible efficiency.

How Fit Should You Be?

Heredity and health determine the top limits to which your physical

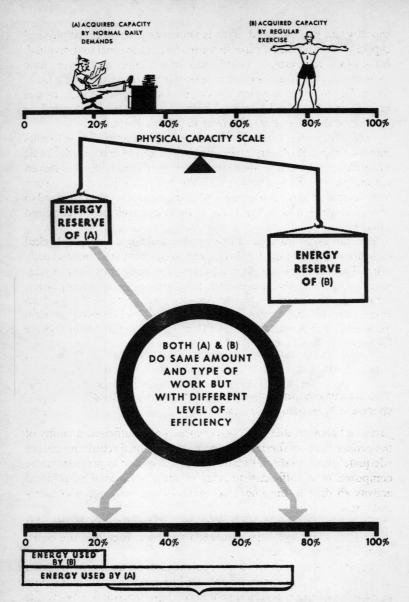

The amount of extra energy left over to enjoy recreational activities by an individual (B) who takes regular exercise

capacity can be developed. This is known as your potential physical capacity. This potential capacity varies from individual to individual. Most of us, for example, could train for a lifetime and never come close to running a four-minute mile simply because we weren't 'built' for it. The top level at which you can perform physically right now is called your 'acquired capacity' because it has been acquired or developed through physical activity in your daily routines.

Your body, like a car, functions most efficiently well below its acquired capacity. A car, for example, driven at its top speed of, say, 110 miles per hour uses more petrol per mile than when it is driven around 50–60 miles per hour, which is well below its capacity. Your body functions in the same way, in that the ratio of work performed to energy expended is better when it functions well below acquired capacity.

You can avoid wastage of energy by acquiring a level of physical capacity well above the level required to perform your normal daily tasks. This can be accomplished by supplementing your daily physical activity with a balanced exercise programme performed regularly. Your capacity increases as you progressively increase the load on your muscular and organic systems. Exercise will increase physical endurance and stamina thus providing a greater reserve of energy for leisure-time activities.

The Contribution of Sports and Other Activities to Basic Physical Efficiency

Just as a balanced diet must be composed of a sufficient quantity of the proper kinds of foods to ensure that nutritional requirements are adequately met, so should a balanced physical activity programme be composed of a sufficient quantity of the proper kind of physical activity so that all the important parts of the body are adequately exercised.

The parts of the body that require special attention are the muscles of the shoulders and arms, abdomen and back, legs, and the heart, lungs, and blood vessels.

No single sport provides a truly balanced development for all parts of the body. This can only be acquired by regular participation in a number of carefully selected sports. Such participation, however, is not possible for the average person for a number of reasons – availability of play opportunity, time, expense. The most practical

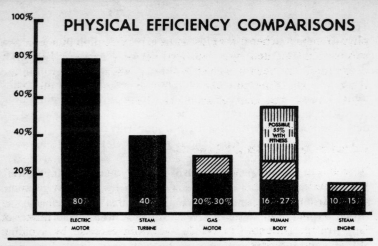

PHYSICAL EFFICIENCY COMPARISONS

		POSSIBLE 55% WITH FITNESS	

80% ELECTRIC MOTOR
40% STEAM TURBINE
20%-30% GAS MOTOR
16%-27% HUMAN BODY
10%-15% STEAM ENGINE

The efficiency of the human body compares poorly with the modern machine. However, through regular exercise its efficiency can be considerably increased

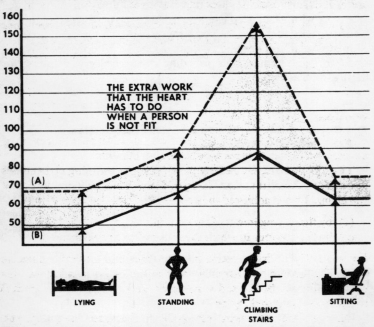

THE EXTRA WORK THAT THE HEART HAS TO DO WHEN A PERSON IS NOT FIT

(A)

(B)

LYING   STANDING   CLIMBING STAIRS   SITTING

This graph illustrates the number of heart-beats required for different routine activities by a human being, (A) before and (B) after a regular vigorous exercise programme

physical fitness scheme for most of us is participation in one or two sports supplemented by a balanced set of exercises. The 5BX programme has been designed to bring physical fitness within the reach of any healthy man who is willing to devote eleven minutes a day to a simple but balanced set of exercises.

Common Sense About Exercise

'It won't do you any good to exercise unless you do it until it hurts', the saying goes. This is absolutely false. Although you may get some benefit from doing exercises until 'it hurts', this is not necessary in order to acquire an adequate level of physical fitness. As a matter of fact, greater benefits can be derived from exercise by avoiding stiffness and soreness.

There are basically two ways in which you can avoid discomfort and still develop high levels of physical capacity:

(1) warm up properly before participating in any strenuous physical activity such as sprinting, handball, tennis, etc.;
(2) start any training programme at a low level of activity and work up by easy stages.

Warming Up

The 5BX Plan was designed so that no additional warm-up is necessary in order to receive its maximum benefits.

The older one is, the more necessary proper warming up becomes to avoid 'strained' muscles. The 5BX Plan has a built-in method of warm-up. This is achieved in two ways:

(1) by the arrangement of the exercises; and
(2) by the manner in which these exercises are performed.

For example the first exercise is a stretching and loosening exercise which limbers up the large muscles of the body. In addition, this exercise should be started very slowly and easily, with a gradual increase in speed and vigour.

Let us see how this principle applies to Exercise One (see p. 26), which requires you to touch the floor. You should not force yourself to do it on the first attempt, but rather start by pushing down very gently and slowly as far as you can without undue strain – then on each succeeding try push down a little harder, and, at the same time, do the exercise a little faster so that by the end of two minutes you are touching the floor and moving at the necessary speed. All the exercises can be performed in this manner.

If you choose to do the exercises in the morning, and are a slow starter, as soon as the alarm rings, stretch, arch your back, lift your legs, and start riding your bicycle.

What is the 5BX Plan?

The 5BX Plan is composed of six charts arranged in progression. Each chart is composed of five exercises which are always performed in the same order and in the same maximum time limit, but, as you progress from chart to chart, there are slight changes in each basic exercise with a gradual demand for more effort.

A sample rating scale of Chart Three is reproduced opposite and is to be used in the following way:

Level These are the physical capacity levels, each indicated by a letter of the alphabet.

Exercises Exercises One, Two, Three, and Four apply to the first four exercises described and illustrated on the following pages. The column headed 1 represents Exercise One (toe touch), etc. The figures in each column indicate the number of times that each exercise is to be repeated in the time allotted for that exercise. Exercise Five is running on the spot. Two activities may be substituted for it, however, and if you prefer you may run or walk the recommended distance in the required time in place of the stationary run of Exercise Five.

Minutes for Each Exercise The allotted time for each exercise is noted at the bottom of the exercise columns. These times remain the same throughout all the charts. Total time for Exercises One to Five is eleven minutes.

Note: It is important that the exercises at any level be completed in eleven minutes. *However, it is likely that in the early stages, an individual will complete certain exercises in less than the allotted time while others may require longer.* In these circumstances the times allotted for individual exercises may be varied within the total eleven-minute period.

Chart 3 Physical capacity rating scale

Level	Exercise					Minutes for: 1 mile run	2 mile walk
	1	**2**	**3**	**4**	**5**		
A+	30	32	47	24	550	8	25
A	30	31	45	22	540	8	25
A−	30	30	43	21	525	8	25
B+	28	28	41	20	510	8¼	28
B	28	27	39	19	500	8¼	26
B−	28	26	37	18	490	8¼	26
C+	26	25	35	17	480	8½	27
C	26	24	34	17	465	8½	27
C−	26	23	33	16	450	8½	27
D+	24	22	31	15	430	8¾	28
D	24	21	30	15	415	8¾	28
D−	24	20	29	15	400	8¾	29
Minutes for each exercise	2	1	1	1	6		

AGE GROUPS

12 yrs maintains D+
13 yrs maintains C+
14 yrs maintains B+

35–9 yrs maintains B
40–44 yrs maintains C

Flying crew 40–44 yrs maintains A+
45–9 yrs maintains B

How Far Should You Progress?

The level of physical capacity to which you should progress is determined by your 'age group'. Levels for flying crew (peak physical fitness) are listed separately. The levels in this plan are based on the expectation of average individuals, and this means there will be some men who are capable of progressing beyond the level indicated, and, on the other hand, there will be persons who will never attain this average level.

Use the goals as guides, and apply them with common sense.

Here Are a Few Tips

When you start, defeat the first desire to skip a day; then defeat all such desires as they occur. This exercise programme has plenty of bite; the longer you do it the more you will enjoy it.

As you progress well into the programme you may find certain levels almost impossible to complete in eleven minutes – but work hard at that level (it may take some days or even weeks) and suddenly you will find yourself sailing ahead again.

Counting the steps in Exercise Five can be difficult. You can lose count very easily at times. If you have this problem, here is an easy way to overcome it. Divide the total number of steps required by seventy-five and note the answer – place a row of buttons, corresponding in number to this answer, on a handy table or chair. Now count off your first seventy-five steps – do your ten required movements – and move the first button. Repeat until all the buttons have been removed, finishing up with any left-over steps. For diversity, occasionally an exercise from the previous chart may be substituted.

How To Begin

Check your daily schedule and determine the time most convenient for you to do the exercises. It should be the same time each day.

Here are some suggested times:

(1) before breakfast;
(2) late morning or afternoon, at your place of employment;
(3) after your regular recreational period;
(4) in the evening just before you retire.

Regardless of the time you choose *start today*.

Maximum Rate of Progression Through Chart One

20 years or under, at least one day at each level
20–29 years, at least two days at each level
30–39 years, at least four days at each level

40–49 years, at least seven days at each level
50–59 years, at least eight days at each level
60 years and over, at least ten days at each level

(If you feel stiff or sore, or if you are unduly breathless at any time, ease up and slow down your rate of progression. This is particularly applicable to the older age groups.)

A Note of Caution

Even if you feel able to start at a high level and progress at a faster rate than indicated – *don't do it* – start at the bottom of Chart One and work up from level to level as recommended.

For best results from 5BX the exercises must be done *regularly*. Remember, it may take you, 6, 8, 10 months or more of daily exercises to attain the level recommended for you, but once you have attained it, only three periods of exercise per week will maintain this level of physical capacity. If for any reason (illness, etc.) you stop doing 5BX regularly and you wish to begin again, *do not* recommence at the level you had attained previously.

Do drop back several levels until you find one you can do without undue strain. After a period of inactivity of longer than two months, or one month if caused by illness, it is recommended that you start again at Chart One.

How to Progress

Start at the lowest physical capacity level of Chart One (D –). Repeat each exercise in the allotted time or do the five exercises in eleven minutes. Move upwards on the same chart to the next level, D, only after you can complete all the required movements at your present level within eleven minutes. Continue to progress upwards in this manner until you can complete all the required movements at level A + within eleven minutes. Now start at the bottom of Chart Two (D –), and continue in this fashion upwards through the levels, and from chart to chart, until you reach the level for your age group; e.g. age 35–9 (B Chart Three) does 32 levels from D – on Chart One to B on Chart Three.

Chart 1 Physical capacity rating scale

Level	Exercise					Minutes for: ½ mile run	1 mile walk
	1	2	3	4	5		
A+	20	18	22	13	400	5½	17
A	18	17	20	12	375	5½	17
A−	16	15	18	11	335	5½	17
B+	14	13	16	9	320	6	18
B	12	12	14	8	305	6	18
B−	10	11	12	7	280	6	18
C+	8	9	10	6	260	6½	19
C	7	8	9	5	235	6½	19
C−	6	7	8	4	205	6½	19
D+	4	5	6	3	175	7	20
D	3	4	5	3	145	7½	21
D−	2	3	4	2	100	8	21
Minutes for each exercise	2	1	1	1	6		

AGE GROUPS

6 yrs maintains B

7 yrs maintains A

1

Feet astride, arms upward.

Forward bend to floor touching then stretch upward and backward bend.

Do not strain to keep knees straight.

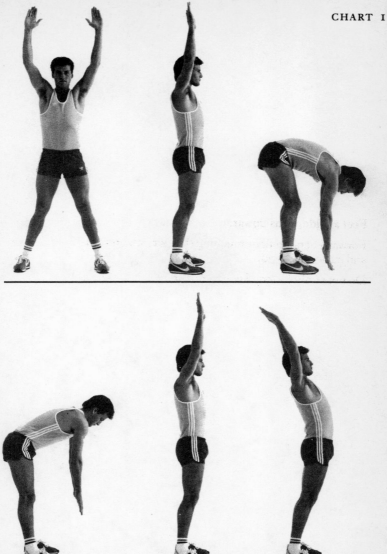

27

2

Back lying, feet 6 ins. apart, arms at sides.

Sit up just far enough to see your heels.

Keep legs straight, head and shoulders must clear the floor.

CHART I

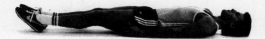

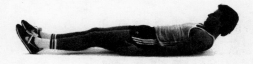

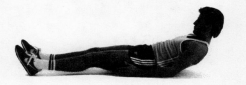

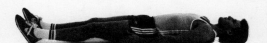

2

3

Front lying, palms placed under the thighs.

Raise head and one leg, repeat using legs alternately.

Keep leg straight at the knee, thighs must clear the palms.

(Count one each time second leg touches floor.)

CHART I

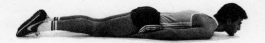

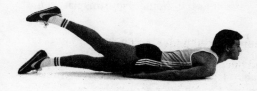

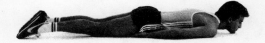

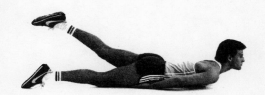

3

4

Front lying, hands under the shoulders, palms flat on the floor.

Straighten arms lifting upper body, keeping the knees on the floor. Bend arms to lower body.

Keep body straight from the knees, arms must be fully extended, chest must touch floor to complete one movement.

CHART I

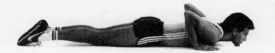

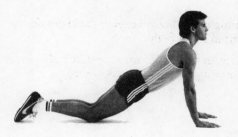

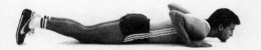

4

5 Stationary run

(Count a step each time left foot touches floor.)

Lift feet approximately 4 ins. off floor.

Every 75 steps do 10 'scissor jumps'.

Repeat this sequence until required number of steps
is completed.

Scissor jumps

Stand with right leg and left arm extended forward, and
left leg and right arm extended backward.

Jump up – change position of arms and legs before
landing.

Repeat (arms shoulder high).

CHART I

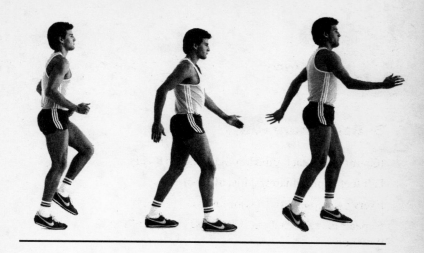

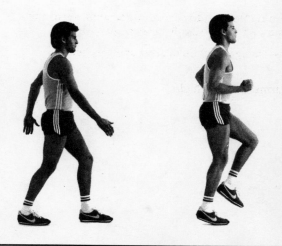

5

Chart 2 Physical capacity rating scale

Level	Exercise					Minutes for:	
	1	2	3	4	5	1 mile run	2 mile walk
A+	30	23	33	20	500	9	30
A	29	21	31	19	485	9	31
A−	28	20	29	18	470	9	32
B+	26	18	27	17	455	9½	33
B	24	17	25	16	445	9½	33
B−	22	16	23	15	440	9½	33
C+	20	15	21	14	425	10	34
C	19	14	19	13	410	10	34
C−	18	13	17	12	395	10	34
D+	16	12	15	11	380	10½	35
D	15	11	14	10	360	10½	35
D−	14	10	13	9	335	10½	35
Minutes for each exercise	2	1	1	1	6		

AGE GROUPS

8 yrs maintains D −
9 yrs maintains C −
10 yrs maintains B −
11 yrs maintains A −

45−9 yrs maintains A +
50−60 yrs maintains C +

1

Feet astride, arms upward.

Touch floor and press (bounce) once then stretch upward and backward bend.

Do not strain to keep knees straight.

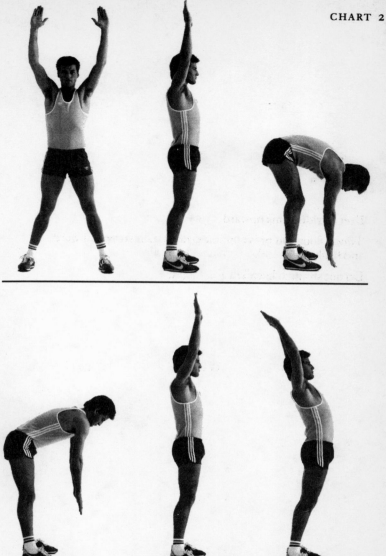

CHART 2

1

2

Back lying, feet 6 ins. apart, arms at sides.

'Sit up' to vertical position, keep feet on floor even if it is necessary to hook them under a chair.

Allow knees to bend slightly.

CHART 2

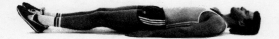

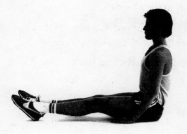

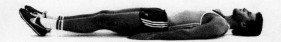

2

3

Front lying, palms placed under thighs.

Raise head, shoulders, and both legs.

Keep legs straight, both thighs must clear the palms.

CHART 2

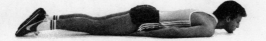

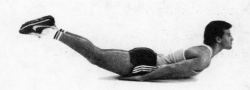

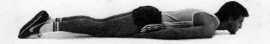

3

4

Front lying, hands under the shoulders, palms flat on floor.

Straighten arms to lift body with only palms and toes on the floor. Back straight.

Chest must touch floor for each completed movement after arms have been fully extended.

CHART 2

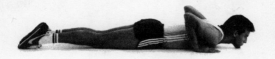

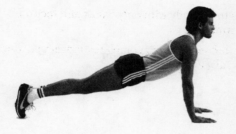

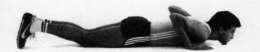

4

5 Stationary run

(Count a step each time left foot touches floor.)

Lift feet approximately 4 ins. off floor.

After every 75 steps, do 10 'astride jumps'.

Repeat this sequence until required number of steps
is completed.

Astride jumps

Feet together, arms at side.

Jump and land with feet astride and arms raised sideways
to slightly above shoulder height.

Return with a jump to the starting position for count of
one. Keep arms straight.

CHART 2

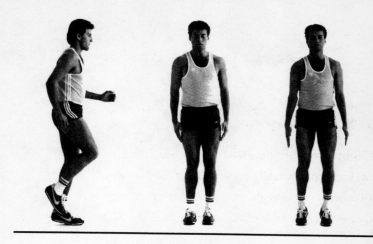

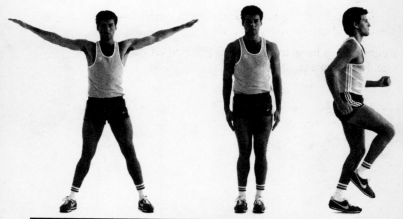

5

Chart 3 Physical capacity rating scale

Level	Exercise					Minutes for: 1 mile run	2 mile walk
	1	**2**	**3**	**4**	**5**		
A+	30	32	47	24	550	8	25
A	30	31	45	22	540	8	25
A−	30	30	43	21	525	8	25
B+	28	28	41	20	510	8¼	28
B	28	27	39	19	500	8¼	26
B−	28	26	37	18	490	8¼	26
C+	26	25	35	17	480	8½	27
C	26	24	34	17	465	8½	27
C−	26	23	33	16	450	8½	27
D+	24	22	31	15	430	8¾	28
D	24	21	30	15	415	8¾	28
D−	24	20	29	15	400	8¾	29
Minutes for each exercise	2	1	1	1	6		

AGE GROUPS

12 yrs maintains D+
13 yrs maintains C+
14 yrs maintains B+

35–9 yrs maintains B
40–44 yrs maintains C

Flying crew 40–44 yrs maintains A+
45–9 yrs maintains B

1

Feet astride, arms upward.

Touch floor 6 ins. outside left foot, again between feet and press once, then 6 ins. outside right foot, bend backward as far as possible, repeat, reverse direction after half the number of counts.

Do not strain to keep knees straight, return to erect position.

CHART 3

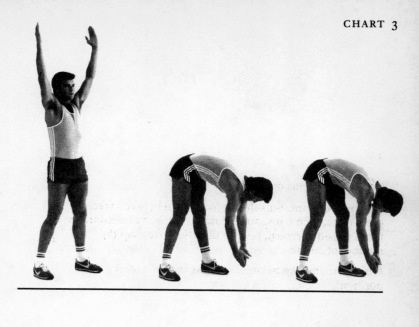

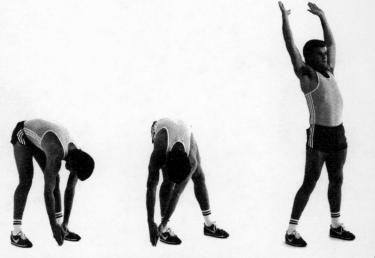

1

2

Back lying, feet 6 ins. apart, arms clasped behind head.

Sit up to vertical position, keep feet on floor, hook feet under chair, etc., only if necessary.

CHART 3

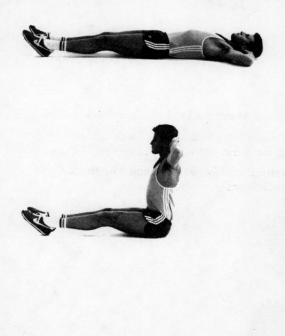

3

Front lying, hands interlocked behind the back.

Lift head, shoulders, chest, and both legs as high as possible.

Keep legs straight, and raise chest and both thighs completely off floor.

CHART 3

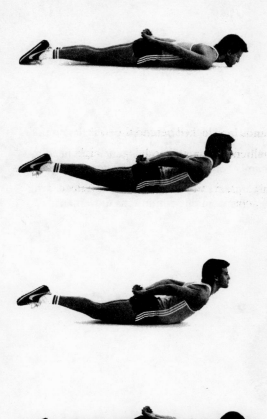

4

Front lying, hands under the shoulders, palms flat on floor.

Touch chin to floor in front of hands – touch forehead to floor behind hands before returning to up position.

There are three definite movements, chin, forehead, arms straightened. *Do not do* in one continuous movement.

CHART 3

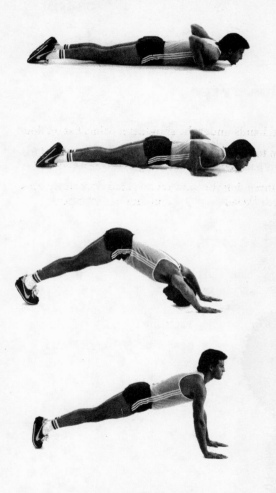

4

5 Stationary run

(Count a step each time left foot touches floor.)

Lift feet approximately 4 ins. off floor.

After every 75 steps do 10 'half knee bends'.

Repeat this sequence until required number of steps is completed.

Half knee bends

Feet together, hands on hips, knees bent to form an angle of about 110 degrees; do not bend knees past a right angle.

Straighten to upright position, raising heels off floor, return to starting position each time.

Keep feet in contact with floor – the back upright and straight at all times.

CHART 3

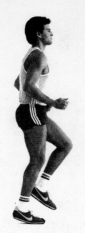 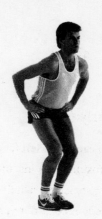

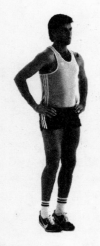 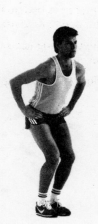 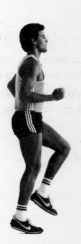

5

Chart 4 Physical capacity rating scale

| Level | Exercise | | | | | Minutes for: | |
	1	2	3	4	5	1 mile run	2 mile walk
A+	30	22	50	42	400	7	19
A	30	22	49	40	395	7	19
A−	30	22	49	37	390	7	19
B+	28	21	47	34	380	7¼	20
B	28	21	46	32	375	7¼	20
B−	28	21	46	30	365	7¼	20
C+	26	19	44	28	355	7½	21
C	26	19	43	26	345	7½	21
C−	26	19	43	24	335	7½	21
D+	24	18	41	21	325	7¾	23
D	24	18	40	19	315	7¾	23
D−	24	18	40	17	300	7¾	23
Minutes for each exercise	2	1	1	1	6		

AGE GROUPS

15 yrs maintains D −
16–17 yrs maintains C +

25–9 yrs maintains A +
30–34 yrs maintains C −

Flying crew   30–34 yrs maintains B
35–9 yrs maintains C −

1

Feet astride, arms upward.

Touch floor outside left foot, between feet, press once, then outside right foot, circle, bend backward as far as possible, reverse directions after half the number of counts.

Do not strain to keep knees straight.

Keep arms above head and make full circle, bending backward past vertical each time.

CHART 4

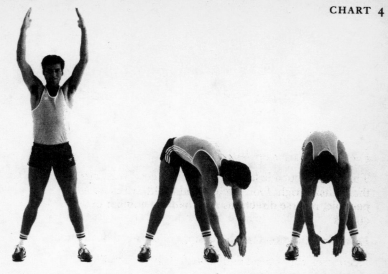

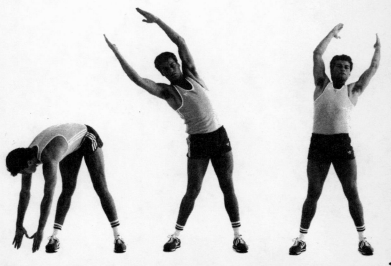

2

Back lying, legs straight, feet together, arms straight overhead.

Sit up and touch the toes keeping the arms and legs straight. Use chair to hook feet under only if necessary.

Keep arms in contact with the sides of the head throughout the movement.

Allow knees to bend slightly.

CHART 4

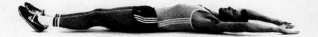

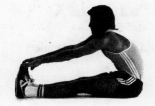

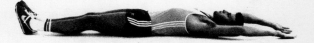

2

3

Front lying, hands and arms stretched sideways.

Lift head, shoulders, arms, chest, and both legs as high as possible.

Keep legs straight, raise chest and both thighs completely off floor.

CHART 4

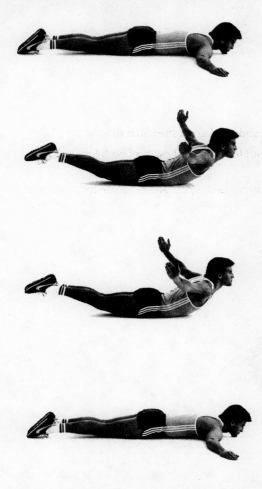

3

4

Front lying, palms of hands flat on floor, approximately
1 foot from ears directly to side of head.

Straighten arms to lift body.

Chest must touch floor for each completed movement.

CHART 4

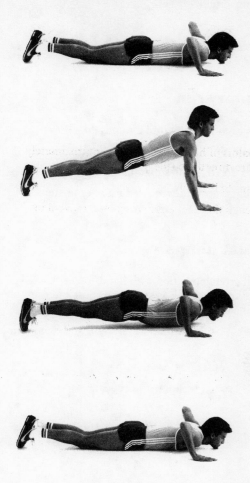

4

5 Stationary run

(Count a step each time left foot touches floor.)

Lift knees waist high.

Every 75 steps do 10 'semi-squat jumps'.

Repeat this sequence until required number of steps
is completed.

Semi-squat jumps

Drop to a half crouch position with hands on knees and
arms straight, keeping back as straight as possible, right
foot slightly ahead of left.

Jump to upright position with body straight and feet leaving
floor.

Reverse position of feet before landing.

Return to half crouch position and repeat.

CHART 4

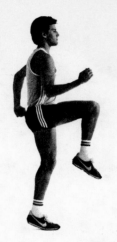
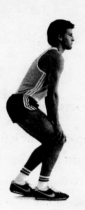
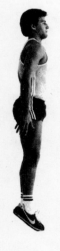
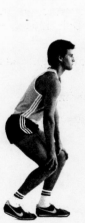
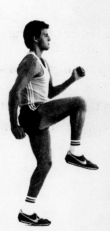

5

Chart 5 Physical capacity rating scale

Level	Exercise					Mins:Secs for 1 mile run
	1	2	3	4	5	
A+	30	40	50	44	500	6:00
A	30	39	49	43	485	6:06
A−	30	38	48	42	475	6:09
B+	28	36	47	40	465	6:12
B	28	35	46	39	455	6:15
B−	28	34	45	38	445	6:21
C+	26	32	44	36	435	6:27
C	26	31	43	35	420	6:33
C−	26	30	42	34	410	6:39
D+	24	28	41	32	400	6:45
D	24	27	40	31	385	6:51
D−	24	26	39	30	375	7:00
Minutes for each exercise	2	1	1	1	6	

AGE GROUPS

18–25 yrs maintains C   *Flying crew*   Under 25 yrs maintains B+
25–9 yrs maintains D+

1

Feet astride, arms upward, hands clasped, arms straight.

Touch floor outside left foot, between feet, press once, then outside right foot, circle bend backward as far as possible.

Reverse direction after half the number of counts.

Do not strain to keep knees straight.

CHART 5

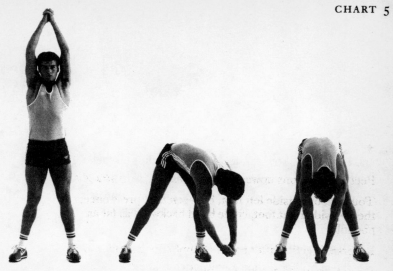

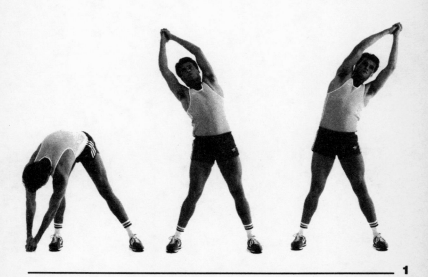

1

2

Back lying, legs straight, feet together, hands clasped behind head.

Sit up and raise legs in bent position, at same time twist to touch right elbow to left knee. This completes one movement.

Alternate the direction of twist each time.

Keep feet off floor when elbow touches knee.

CHART 5

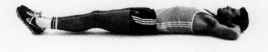

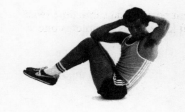

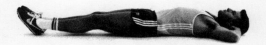

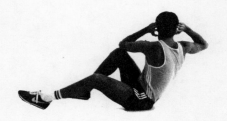

2

3

Front lying, arms extended overhead.

Raise arms, head, chest, and both legs as high as possible.

Keep legs and arms straight, chest and both thighs completely off floor.

CHART 5

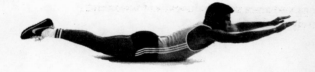

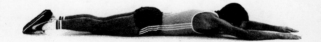

3

4

Front lying, hands under shoulders, palms flat on floor.

Push off floor and clap hands before returning to starting position.

Keep body straight during the entire movement. Hand clap must be heard.

CHART 5

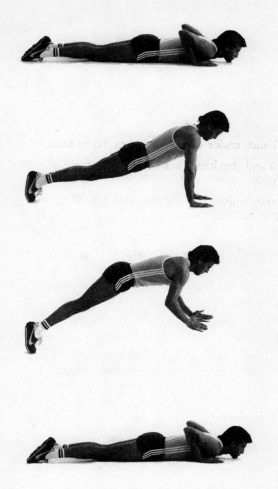

4

5 Stationary run

(Count a step each time left foot touches floor.)

Lift knees waist high.

Every 75 steps do 10 'semi-spread eagle jumps'.

Repeat this sequence until required number of steps is completed.

Semi-spread eagle jumps

Feet together, drop to a half crouch position hands on knees with arms straight.

Jump up to feet astride, swing arms overhead in mid air, return directly to starting position on landing.

Raise hands above head level, spread feet at least shoulder width apart in astride position before landing with feet together.

CHART 5

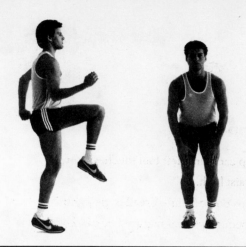

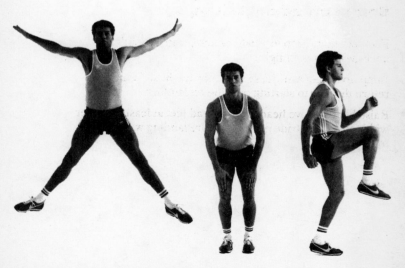

5

Chart 6 Physical capacity rating scale

| Level | Exercise | | | | | Mins:Secs for 1 mile run |
	1	2	3	4	5	
A+	30	50	40	40	600	5:00
A	30	48	39	39	580	5:03
A−	30	47	38	38	555	5:09
B+	28	45	37	36	530	5:12
B	28	44	36	35	525	5:18
B−	28	43	35	34	515	5:24
C+	26	41	34	32	505	5:27
C	26	40	33	31	495	5:33
C−	26	39	32	30	485	5:39
D+	24	37	31	28	475	5:45
D	24	36	30	27	460	5:51
D−	24	35	29	26	450	6:00
Minutes for each exercise	2	1	1	1	6	

Physical capacities in this chart are usually found
only in champion athletes

1

Feet astride, arms upward, hands reverse clasped, arms straight.

Touch floor outside left foot, between feet, press once, then outside right foot, circle bend backwards as far as possible.

Reverse direction after half the number of counts.

Keep hands tightly reverse clasped at all times.

CHART 6

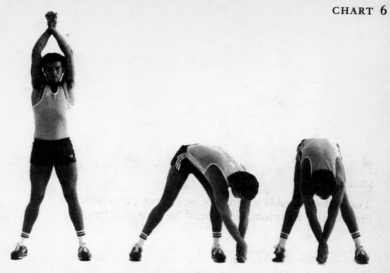

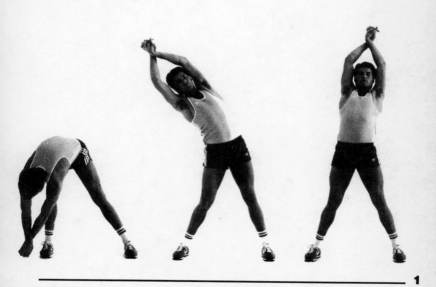

1

2

Back lying, legs straight, feet together, arms straight over the head.

Sit up and at the same time lift both legs to touch the toes in a pike (V) position.

Keep feet together, legs and arms straight, all of the upper back and legs clear floor, fingers touch toes each time.

CHART 6

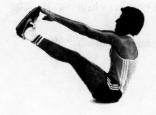

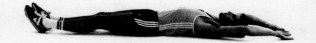

2

3

Front lying, arms extended over head.

Raise arms, head, chest, and both legs as high as possible then press back once.

Keep legs and arms straight – chest and both thighs completely off floor.

CHART 6

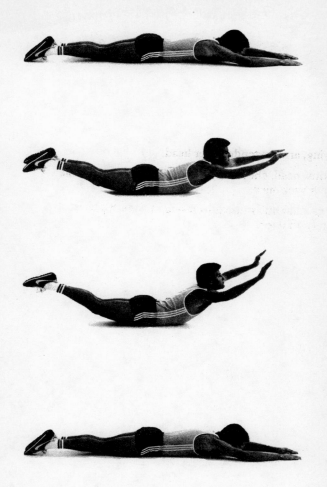

4

Front lying, hands under shoulders, palms flat on floor.

Push off floor and slap chest before returning to starting position.

Keep body straight during the entire movement, chest slap must be heard.

CHART 6

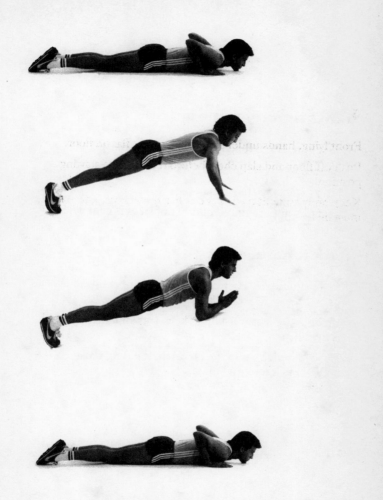

_____ **4**

5 Stationary run

(Count a step each time left foot touches floor.)

Lift knees waist high.

Every 75 steps do 10 'jack jumps'.

Repeat this until required number of steps is completed.

Jack jumps

Feet together, knees bent. Sit on heels, finger tips touch floor.

Jump up, raise legs waist high, keep legs straight and touch toes in mid air.

Keep legs straight, raise feet level to 'standing waist height'. Touch toes each time.

CHART 6

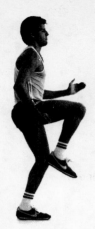

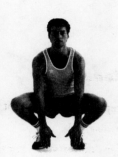

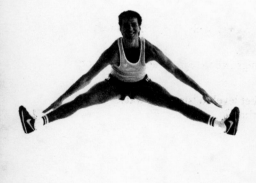

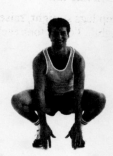

5